LOSING WEIGHT THE AFRICAN WAY

LOSING WEIGHT THE AFRICAN WAY

D'Maye

ISBN 978-1-300-86417-2

Introduction

Congratulations. This is probably the last book you will ever need to read on how to lose weight. I am convinced if you follow the diet and exercise program outlined in this book, you will see the weight fall off and disappear for good.

Disclaimer

The information and materials contained in this book are the personal views and experiences of the author and is not a substitute for medical advice and therapy. It should be used only as a guide. Always consult a qualified fitness professional before attempting any new exercise regime or unfamiliar move.

The author specifically disclaims liability, loss or risk personal or otherwise, that is incurred as a consequence, directly or indirectly, from the use or application of any of the contents of this book.

The information contained in this book cannot be used or reproduced by any person or company without being purchased for a fee from or having the written consent of the author. Any unauthorized reproduction is subject to legal action. Any concerns as to the legality of reproduction should be directed to:

The Legal Dept.,
Adesoye Holdings Limited,
Igbonna Road, Offa, Kwara, Nigeria.
Tel: (234) 805-2459778.
E-mail: gmd@adesoyeholdings.com.

About the Author

I am married with three children. My dad is diabetic and I am the eldest of four children. We loved our meals. We could chomp and chew our way through anything. I was not always fat. In fact, I was a skinny kid. Then somewhere in my teens, my appetite kicked in and went into overdrive. I transformed almost overnight from the skinny kid to the fat kid on the block, and I remained that way for most of my young life. I woke up twenty years later and discovered I had high blood pressure and that I was tipping the scales at 115 kg (253lbs), snoring, heavy and sweaty.

"I weighed more than two bags of Cement."

My doctor sang me the same song, he has been singing for a while: *"You need to lose some weight. You have a history of diabetes in your family. You need to exercise more."*

Losing weight was difficult as most of my Nigerian meals were filled to the max with calorie-adding starch and carbohydrates. Meals like Eyan (pounded yam), Eba (dried grated cassava flour), fufu (maize flour), rice, fried plantains, yams, were combined with palm oil-enriched stews.

Typical breakfast was fried eggs, fried yams, bread and butter, baked beans, bacon, sausages or fried potatoes, boiled yams and stew, tea or coffee in the mornings. Then I was off to work. My job required me to sit for long hours, having meetings and punching away at my computer. At eleven, I usually started feeling hungry so I'd have some more tea or coffee or some orange juice. Lunch was a proper meal—my motto was "Anything goes."

I eat as I drink. I tend to swallow my food more than chew, a bad habit of mine and most Nigerian foods are better swallowed than chewed. All drowned with a bottle of my favourite carbonated soft or malt drink. I would eat dinner at about 8.00 or 9.00 p.m. Dinner was also like lunch, anything goes. Then I watched some television, engaged in some social activity or did some more work until I was ready to go to bed. If I felt hungry I ate. I like the feeling of being full. In fact, I was not sure I could sleep on an empty stomach.

I did try to exercise. I tried jogging and bicycling, which I found boring. I loved table tennis and volleyball but it was difficult getting partners. Whenever I thought I'd found my weekly exercise routine, an out of station assignment broke up my routine and by the time I returned, I'd have lost all interests. Also, when I am out of my station, I survive on junk food.

When I tipped the scales at one hundred and fifteen kilograms (253lbs), I knew I needed to do something fast. And so began my attempts at loosing losing weight.

MY FIRST ATTEMPT (LUNCH AND DINNER ONLY DIET)

I skipped breakfast in the mornings because it made me groggy anyway, so I have a cup of tea or coffee with milk and sugar. At eleven I usually started feeling hungry so I'd have some more tea or coffee or some packaged flavoured juice. Lunch and dinner was a mix of carbohydrate and starchy foods with all the trimmings. After the meal, I would usually need a nap. THE RESULT: *There was no change in my weight.*

SECOND ATTEMPT (NO MORE LUNCH DIET)

For breakfast and because I did not want to feel groggy, I would have some cereal with milk and some sugar. For brunch I could have some tea or coffee with sugar and milk or some packaged flavoured fruit juice or sweetened yogurt. I would then skip lunch and wait for dinner. Since dinner was my only proper meal of the day, I will reward myself with a proper and filling meal. THE RESULTS: *There was no change in my weight.*

THIRD ATTEMPT (NO MORE DINNER DIET)

Again I decided to switch things. I would have a light breakfast of grain cereal with milk or just tea, coffee with milk and sugar. If I felt hungry at eleven, I would have some more tea or coffee with brown sugar and powdered milk or some package flavoured juice or unsweetened yogurt. Lunch was still a mix of carbohydrate and starchy foods with all the trimmings and a nap. To help me sleep at night I would have some fruits with plenty of water THE RESULT: *For the first time, I noticed some positive change in my weight.* I continued on this road for a while, adding and removing certain foods in my diet, until I discovered the rules, which saved my life. Today I weigh 90kg (198lbs); my waistline has shrunk from 42" to 34". My dress size dropped from extra-extra large to medium and I am packing lean muscle.

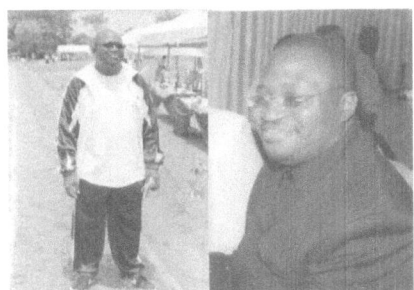
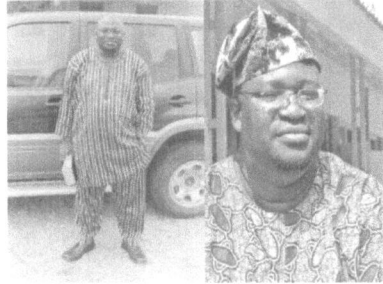
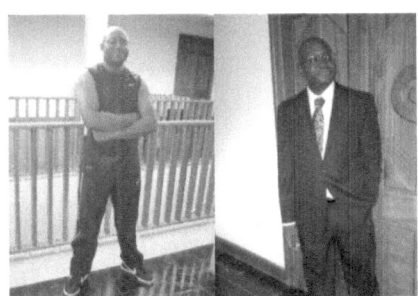
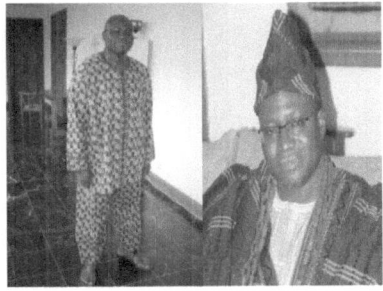

Table of Contents

The Rules

To lose weight my way, you have to play by the rules. There are rules that should never be broken. I call them Solid Rules because they don't change and then there are some rules, which allow you some flexibility; I call those, Liquid Rules. So to lose weight my way requires the combination of both Solid Rules and Liquid Rules.

❖ SOLID RULES

You must exercise in the mornings. Exercise jumpstarts the Metabolism.
When you drink, drink water. Never let yourself get dehydrated. Water keeps the skin supple and get rids of the uric acid that can build up from protein-enriched diets.
It's all about the drinks. Only drink after you finish your meal.
Have breakfast. It helps to start your metabolism. Never go hungry.
Eat your heaviest meal at lunch.
You must stop eating two hours before you sleep.
You must exercise before you sleep. Keeps the fire burning while you sleep.
Use exercise equipment. Variety is the spice of life.
Discover your Body Mass Index (BMI).
Weigh yourself the same way, once every week.

❖ LIQUID RULES

Choose a routine, like squats or jogging with intermittent sprints that will get your heart pumping for at least five minutes.
You may have tea, green tea, herbal tea or coffee without sugar. You may add some powdered milk or natural honey.
Do not eat to be full. If you feel groggy after a meal you have eaten too much.
Some powdered milk. Nuts and dried fruits are very good. If you enjoy a light breakfast, have a protein snack at eleven. A little snack goes a long way.

Let proteins and vegetables be at least 70% of your meals.

It's all about the timing. If you must eat late, eat raw fruits, dried nuts and raw vegetables (No dressing) drink water, green tea or tea without sugar. Then wait at least an hour before jumping into bed.

If you are invited to party, prepare. Party invitations are a trap. If it is late, aim for the raw salad bar or the fruit basket. If it requires drinking, drink soda water or red wine, but do not get drunk. If it is a buffet, go for the proteins from meats and fish and add a stack of vegetables. If you really like the food, ask if you can take it home for the next day's lunch. Eat before you go. Do not arrive hungry, else you may lose control.

The BMI is a guide and varies from race to race. Let your self-confidence and friends be your guides.

Use the same scale every time you weigh yourself. Do it at the same time each week and in the same manner (without clothes).

Wear body shapers and formers under your clothes. Use vibration belts for the belly. Use a massage chair or get a massage. Invest in some equipment or gym membership.

If the weight is not dropping, change something. It's an evolution. If in two weeks you are not losing more weight or your weight is stagnant, move from a beginner's diet and exercise program to a more hardcore program.

If you have not done any other workout, choose a routine like squats or jogging with intermittent sprints. Anything to get your heart pumping for at least five minutes before you sleep.

Body Mass Index (BMI)

The BODY MASS INDEX (BMI) provides a simple numeric measure of a person's "fatness" or "thinness," allowing health professionals to discuss over- and under-weight problems more objectively. However, BMI has become controversial because many people, including physicians, have come to rely on its apparent numerical authority for medical diagnosis, but that was never the BMI's purpose.

What the BMI numbers mean:
BMI Below 18.5 is underweight; 18.5–24.9 is normal; 25.0–29.9 is overweight, 30.0 and above is obese. To know your BMI use the following formulae.

SI Units $BMI = mass\ (kg) / height\ (m)^2$

Imperial Units $BMI = mass\ (lb) \times 703 / height\ (in)^2$

Imperial Units BMI= $BMI = mass\ (lb) \times 4.88 / height\ (ft)^2$

Imperial Units BMI= $BMI = mass\ (st) \times 9840 / height\ (in)^2$

Instead of relying absolutely on a BMI reading I prefer you work towards a weight that works for you.

Myths

There are myths about diet and exercise. I believe it is my duty to try and dispel some of those myths.

"THERE ARE NO AFRICAN FOODS THAT ONE CAN EAT TO CONTROL ONE'S WEIGHT."

FALSE. There are African foods that are nutritious and can help you lose weight.

"DIETS ARE TOO EXPENSIVE. I CANNOT AFFORD ALL THOSE SUPPLEMENTS."

FALSE. You do not need to spend a fortune on food supplements and drugs.

"YOU DO NOT NEED TO EXERCISE AT ALL TO LOSE WEIGHT."

TRUE. But exercise helps to tone your muscles and skin.

"TO LOSE WEIGHT I ONLY NEED TO EAT ONE PROPER MEAL A DAY."

FALSE. You can eat up to six meals a day and still lose weight. It depends on what you are eating. Eating one meal a day is not healthy, and it may cause your body to think you are starving and therefore refuse to burn fat. It can also cause you to overeat when you eat your one meal for the day.

"TO LOSE WEIGHT I NEED TO STOP EATING MEATS."

FALSE. Except directed by your doctor, meats are full of proteins, and they help maintain your muscles and body systems. The body takes only what it needs from proteins and excretes the rest, unlike carbohydrates and sugars where the excess is stored as fat.

"TO LOSE WEIGHT I NEED TO EAT ONLY VEGETABLES."

FALSE. Though vegetables are low in calories, rich in vitamins and micronutrients you can lose weight by eating other things as well.

"LOSING WEIGHT INVOLVES FEELING HUNGRY."

FALSE. Being hungry is the worst way to diet. My system forbids you to be hungry at any point in time.

"I CANNOT LOSE WEIGHT, BECAUSE OF MY GENETICS ROOTS."

FALSE. While genetics does affect our body types, anyone can lose weight on my diet regardless of genetics.

"MY LIFESTYLE DOES NOT ALLOW ME TO FOLLOW A DIET."

FALSE. You can lose weight on my diet in spite of your lifestyle.

"MY LIFESTYLE DOES NOT ALLOW ME TIME TO EXERCISE."

FALSE. Anyone can exercise, you can do simple exercises as you go about.

"I CAN LOSE WEIGHT BY EATING ANYTHING PROVIDED IT IS IN SMALL. QUANTITIES."

FALSE. If you continue to eat the wrong things, you will eventually get fat.

"SOME PEOPLE ARE JUST MEANT TO BE FAT."

FALSE. People become fat because of their lifestyle and eating habits. If you change these two things you will lose weight.

"MY PARTNER DOES NOT MIND MY BEING OVERWEIGHT."

FALSE. Often our partners love us too much to tell us the truth. You may need to ask someone else for a sincere report.

"BEING OVERWEIGHT HAS NO EFFECT ON ME AT ALL."

FALSE. It is affecting a lot of things in your body, which may tell later on in life.

"ONLY POOR PEOPLE ARE SLIM."

FALSE. Being overweight is not proof of prosperity.

"I AM SLIM SO I AM OKAY."

FALSE. You may be slim because you don't eat properly but that does not make you healthy. Being underweight is also a health risk.

"A LITTLE WEIGHT IS ALLOWED AFTER ONE GETS MARRIED."

FALSE. Your partner married a person as well as an image. When the image changes, it is going to affect your partner's desires towards you, whether your partner admits it or not.

"A LITTLE WEIGHT IS ALLOWED AFTER HAVING CHILDREN."

FALSE. Children are the greatest blessing and the greatest strain on a relationship. Most men begin to cheat at this point, especially if he is still keeping trim and fit. So lose that baby fat.

"I CAN EAT WHAT I LIKE AS LONG AS I EXERCISE AFTERWARDS."

FALSE. Eventually you will eat more than you can burn, especially as you get older, so the weight will just pile up.

"ALCOHOL AND SPIRITS HELPS ME KEEP MY WEIGHT DOWN."

FALSE. Do not think you are doing a good job of controlling your weight by destroying your liver and becoming an alcoholic.

"SMOKING KEEPS ME FROM BEING HUNGRY, SO I SMOKE TO KEEP MY WEIGHT DOWN."

TRUE. But do not think you are doing a good job of controlling your weight by destroying your lungs and becoming an addict.

"ALL DIETS ARE TOO HARD."

FALSE. Not this diet.

"CARDIO AND AEROBIC EXERCISES ARE THE ONLY WAY TO LOSE WEIGHT."

FALSE. There are other forms of exercise that can burn fat for longer periods than cardio or aerobics.

"I CAN EAT WHAT I LIKE PROVIDED I DRINK A DIETER'S TEA OR SUPPLEMENT THAT WILL STOP MY SYSTEM FROM ABSORBING THE FOOD AFTERWARDS."

TRUE. But regardless of what you drink or swallow afterwards there is a price to pay for not eating right.

"ALL I NEED ARE PILLS THAT BURN FAT."

FALSE. Remember that all pills have some side effects. Also, pills will not tone your muscles.

"ALL I NEEDS IS SOME OF THOSE SLIMMING FOODS."

FALSE. Most of them are not filling or tasty enough for you to endure while waiting for your weight to drop. And because it can be so restrictive, most people regain the weight the moment they stop. They are also not cheap.

"TO EXERCISE I NEED SOME SERIOUS EQUIPMENT."

FALSE. *You do not have to go overboard buying a lot of fancy and expensive equipment especially when you cannot afford it. Most exercises have natural (equipment-free) alternatives. Equipment, however, may help to give variety and colour to exercise routines, which ordinarily can become less motivating after a while. So a combination of equipment and non-equipment-based exercises works best.*

"WHEN YOU START TO EXERCISE YOUR FAMILY AND FRIENDS WILL SUPPORT YOU."

FALSE. *Be prepared to go on regardless of support or not. Also family and friends may not know how to push you to excel, because they love you so much.*

"WHEN YOU START TO TRY TO EAT RIGHT YOUR FAMILY AND FRIENDS WILL HELP YOU."

FALSE. *They may be your greatest temptation, as they gorge themselves in front of you. You may have to fight to eat right.*

"I SHOULD DROP A DRESS SIZE AFTER A WEEK OF DIET AND NUTRITION."

FALSE. *For most people this is not possible. It took time for the weight to pile up and it may take some time to get rid of it.*

"AS A WOMAN, IF I LIFT WEIGHTS I WILL BUILD MUSCLE AND LOOK LIKE A MAN.

FALSE. *There are weight exercises that burn fat only. These exercises firm the muscles that support the breasts, hips, buttocks, the belly and underarms which are usually the problem areas.*

"EATING IS PERSONAL."

TRUE. *People enjoy various foods and some have varying levels of tolerance to different kinds of foods. One rule cannot fit all, which is why our recipes allows you to prepare and combine the listed foods in a way you can enjoy.*

"LOSING WEIGHTS REQUIRES SOME RESEARCH."

TRUE. *A little more information never hurt anyone. To motivate yourself, buy fitness magazines or join a support group. You will learn what exercises and foods works the best for you, using simple guidelines and common sense.*

"LOSING WEIGHT IS NOT FOREVER."

TRUE. *When you achieve your goal you can ease up on some of the restricted foods, As long as your body weight remains unchanged.*

The Warnings

With every good thing, there may be side effects. Please read the following information carefully.

"THIS BOOK MAY IMPROVE YOUR HEART."
TRUE. The exercises included within this book may strengthen your heart.

"THIS BOOK MAY IMPROVE YOUR SEX LIFE."
TRUE. Your inhibitions may drop because you look so good.

"THIS BOOK MAY IMPROVE YOUR SELF IMAGE GIVE YOU SEX APPEAL AND CONFIDENCE."
TRUE. Looking your best always give you self confidence and people will notice.

"THIS BOOK MAY CAUSE A CHANGE IN LIFE STYLE."
TRUE. When the weight begins to come off, you may be motivated to continue to make more healthy choices.

"THIS BOOK MAY MAKE YOU BUY SOME NEW CLOTHES."
TRUE. Your old clothes may no longer fit.

"THIS BOOK MAY CAUSE YOU TO SPEND MONEY ON YOUR APPEARANCE."
TRUE. People will notice you and if commendations keep coming, you may always want to look your best.

"THIS BOOK MAY MAKE YOU LOOK YOUNGER THAN YOUR AGE."
TRUE. Losing weight may make us look younger than our age, while putting on weight can make us look older.

"THIS BOOK MAY CAUSE YOU TO STOP SNORING WHEN YOU SLEEP."
TRUE. If your airways are constricted because of fat.

**"THIS BOOK MAY CAUSE MEMBERS OF THE
OPPOSITE SEX TO NOTICE YOU."**
TRUE. Couples Beware."

"THIS BOOK MAY MAKE YOU PHYSICALLY STRONG."
TRUE. Especially if you do the weight training exercises.

**"THIS BOOK MAY MAKE IT DIFFICULT FOR YOU TO
ENJOY CERTAIN FOODS AND DRINKS AGAIN."**
*TRUE. Once your body begins to eat only natural foods, it may not like the
alternatives and neither will you.*

"THIS BOOK MAY COST YOU SOME FRIENDSHIPS."
*TRUE. You may have to avoid certain places and friends for a while to
survive the diet.*

The Diet Menu

My diet is made up five daily meals so you never go hungry. I recommend everyone start with the Beginner's Diet. The Beginner's Diet will gently ease you into the nutritional benefits of eating right and as the weights falls off and your body adjusts to the regime, you can then proceed to the Intermediate and Hardcore Diets, which are more rigid. The reverse is also true, when you attain your desired weight. You can then ease back from the Hardcore Diet to the Beginner's Diet.

The Beginners Diet

❖ THE BEGINNERS BREAKFAST

Cereal breakfast, milk and sugar
Boiled eggs
Poached eggs
Raw fruits
Raw salad and low-fat dressing
Moin moin (Bean pudding)
Bean cakes (akara)
Grilled chicken
Grilled fish
Grilled turkey
Turkey slices
Chicken slices
Peppered chicken
Peppered meats
Peppered fish
Jollof beans
Fish pepper soup
Chicken pepper soup

Assorted meat pepper soups
Bush meat pepper soups
Goat meat pepper soup
Tea/coffee, milk, sugar
Flat bread
Tomatoes
Onions
Broccoli
Carrots

❖ THE BEGINNERS ELEVENSES

Tea/coffee, milk, sugar
Cold water (with ice)
Sweetened yogurt
Coke Zero (sugar free)
7-up sugar-free
Nutritional bars
Oranges
Pineapples
Bananas
Tangerines
Apples
Kiwi
Pears
Melons
Mangoes
Salad
Dry crackers (Jacob's)
Peppered chicken
Peppered meats
Peppered fish
Beef jerky (kilichi)
Dried Fish (panla)
Suya

❖ THE BEGINNERS LUNCH

Jollof beans
Beans
Moin moin (bean pudding)

Spinach (efo)
Catfish pepper soup
Fish pepper soup
Chicken pepper soup
Cow tail pepper soup
Meat pepper soup
Goat meat pepper soup
Beans stew (gbegiri)
Humus
Rice (cooked, handful only)
Grilled chicken
Grilled fish
Grilled meats
Peppered meats
Peppered fish
Peppered chicken
Tomatoes
Onions
Broccoli
Carrots
Edikang ikong stew
Ogbono stew
Ewudu stew
Okra stew
Mixed vegetable sauce
Stir-fry beans

❖ THE BEGINNER'S TEA (OPTIONAL)

Tea/ coffee, no sugar
Cold water
Natural unsweetened yogurt
Natural nuts (almonds)
Natural nuts (pecans)
Natural seeds (unsalted pumpkin seeds)
Dried mango slices
Beef jerky (kilichi)
Dried fish (kpanla)
Soda water (flavoured)
Dry crackers (Jacob's)

❖ THE BEGINNER'S SUPPER

Oranges
Pineapples
Bananas
Tangerines
Apples
Kiwi
Pears
Melons
Soda water (flavoured)

The Intermediate Diet

❖ THE INTERMEDIATE BREAKFAST

Muesli and powdered milk (no sugar)
Poached eggs
Raw fruits
Raw salad (balsamic vinegar dressing)
Moin moin (bean pudding)
Grilled chicken
Grilled fish
Grilled meats
Peppered chicken
Peppered meats
Peppered fish
Stir-fry beans
Fish pepper soup
Chicken pepper soup
Cowtail pepper soup
Turkey slices
Chicken slices
Tomatoes
Onions
Carrots

❖ THE INTERMEDIATE ELEVENSES

Tea/coffee, milk (no sugar)
Skimmed milk
Honey
Brown sugar
Cold water (with ice)
Natural unsweetened yogurt
Natural nuts (almonds)
Natural nuts (pecans)
Natural nuts (unsalted pumpkin seeds)
Dried mango slices
Beef jerky (kilichi)
Dried fish (kpanla)
Soda water (plain) with natural juices

❖ THE INTERMEDIATE LUNCH

Stir-fry beans
Plain beans
Moin moin (bean pudding)
Salad
Efo
Fish pepper soup
Chicken pepper soup
Cowtail pepper soup
Beans stew (gbegiri)
Humus
Ofada rice (cooked handful only)
Grilled chicken
Grilled fish
Grilled meats
Peppered meats
Peppered fish
Peppered chicken
Tomatoes
Onions
Broccoli
Carrots
Edikang ikong stew

Ogbono stew
Ewudu stew
Okra stew
Mixed vegetable sauce
Stir fry beans

❖ THE INTERMEDIATE TEA (OPTIONAL)

Tea/coffee, milk (no sugar)
Skimmed milk
Honey
Brown sugar
Cold water (with ice)
Natural unsweetened yogurt
Natural nuts (almonds)
Natural nuts (pecans)
Natural nuts (unsalted pumpkin seeds)
Dried mango slices
Beef jerky (kilichi)
Dried fish (kpanla)
Soda water (plain) with natural juices

❖ THE INTERMEDIATE SUPPER

Oranges
Pineapples
Bananas
Tangerines
Apples
Kiwi
Pears
Melons
Soda water (flavoured)

The Hardcore Diet

❖ THE HARDCORE BREAKFAST

Raw fruits, 100%
Jollof beans

Moin moin (bean pudding)
Raw salad
Grilled chicken
Grilled fish
Grilled meats
Poached eggs (no yolk)
Peppered chicken
Peppered meats
Peppered fish
Fish pepper soup
Chicken pepper soup
Cow tail pepper soup
Tomatoes
Onions
Broccoli
Carrots

❖ THE HARDCORE ELEVENSES

Tea/coffee No sugar
Green tea
Cold water (with ice)
Natural unsweetened yogurt
Natural nuts(Almonds)
Natural nuts(Pecans)
Natural nuts (unsalted pumpkin seeds)
Dried mango slices
Beef jerky (kilichi)
Dried fish (kpanla)
Soda water (plain)
Soda water (plain) with natural juices

❖ THE HARDCORE LUNCH

Stir fry beans
Plain beans
Moin moin (bean pudding)
Poached eggs
Fish pepper soup
Chicken pepper soup

Cowtail pepper soup
Meat pepper soup
Spinach (efo)
Beans stew (gbegiri)
Humus
Grilled chicken
Grilled fish
Grilled meats
Peppered chicken
Peppered meats
Peppered fish
Tomatoes
Onions
Broccoli
Carrots
Edikang ikong stew
Ogbono stew
Ewudu stew
Okra stew
Mixed vegetable sauce
Stir fry beans
Tea (optional)
Tea/coffee, no sugar
Green tea
Cold water
Natural unsweetened yogurt
Natural nuts (almonds)
Natural nuts (pecans)
Natural nuts (unsalted pumpkin seeds)
Dried mango slices
Beef jerky (kilichi)
Dried fish (kpanla)
Soda water (plain)
Soda water (plain) with natural juices

❖ THE HARDCORE SUPPER

Bananas
Tangerines
Apples

Kiwi
Pears
Melons
Green tea
Soda water (plain)
Soda water (plain) with natural juices

The African continent is made of a variety of cultures and indigenous foods which means an endless supply of cuisine styles. You will need to build your own menu using the foods that are local to your environment. To help you, please follow these guidelines:

Protein-rich foods are the best.
Avoid fried meats and fried vegetables.
Eat foods grilled or broiled.

Boil or steam meat and vegetables.
Avoid foods rich in carbohydrates and sugars.
Avoid food made from starchy tubers and grains.
Substitute processed foods for natural ones.
Avoid the fatty portions of meats and fish.
Avoid pork.
Eat lean meat portions from wild animals
Avoid foods made with butter, flour, fats, margarine and wines.
Substitute your oils and fats with vegetable oil or olive oil.
Add vegetables to your meals; it helps digestion.
Avoid beer and alcohol.
For desserts, go for fruits, nuts and natural yogurt. No cakes.
Drink lots of water, teas and coffees to help control the proteins.
Avoid canned foods, soups and fruits.
Use nuts, spices and fruits to enhance the flavour of your meals.
For salad, use balsamic vinegar or olive oil as dressing instead of mayonnaise.
Use nuts, seeds and fruits, grilled meat and fish pieces to enhance your salads.
Drink teas and coffee after your meals. They help digestion.
Green tea stops the absorption of fats and can suppress appetite.
Carry a bag of fruits, seeds and nuts with you.
Eggs should be eaten boiled or poached, but not fried.
Avoid bread and pastries, except flat bread and oat bread.
Use unsweetened milk, unflavoured, powdered or skimmed (low fat) milk
Eat four to six small meals, instead of one to three large meals.

No snacking on sweets, chocolates, crisps and chewing gums.
Fruit juices should be natural, avoid flavoured juices loaded with sugars.

To know if you are eating well and exercising right, weigh yourself weekly. Weekly because of issues with water retention and situations caused by hormonal activity. If the weight is dropping then you are eating well. However, if you are no longer losing the weight, do not despair, you may be building lean muscle so move towards the Hardcore Diet or increase your aerobic and cardio exercises. If you still need some guidance, please send me an email at losingweighttheafricanway@yahoo.com. I will do my best to answer your questions.

The Exercise Menu

Exercises help burn the fat calls of the body and tone the skin. If you diet alone without some form of exercise, you will lose weight but it may not be obvious because of the loosening of the skin. Exercises help the skin in contracting to the new you. On the flipside, if you exercise but do not watch your diet, your weight would at best stagnate despite your best effort. This is what happens to pot-bellied individuals who can play sports, but refuse to eat and drink right. The overall effort is wasted.

If you are over forty or have a health condition, you may need to consult your physician before doing any of these exercises. If you are over a 100 kg (220 lbs) you need to be careful when doing cardio and aerobic exercises because of the impact of the weight on your knees and ankles. In this book, we have exercises that can be done daily (cardio and aerobic) and some that should not (fat blasting and toning exercises) and then there are those for adding muscle mass (muscle exercises).

Cardio and Aerobic Exercises

These exercises can be done daily. Start with stretches to warm up the muscles. Use a dance video of your choice. There are many varieties and styles to suit every taste and fitness level. If you like to jog or walk, intersperse your jogs or walk with sprints or jogs. Jog (walk) for 2 minutes. Sprint (jog) for 1 minute. Jog (walk) for another 2 minutes. That completes 1 cycle. Repeat cycles according to your fitness level. Keep it under a maximum of 30 minutes (6 cycles).

Those who don't like to run can engage in any sporting activities they enjoy, provided it raises one's heart rate into the metabolic range (where fat is burned). This is determined by the number of heart beats per minute and varies according to age, height and weight. You can also measure this by counting your pulse. There are a variety of places you can measure your heart rate (pulse), but the easiest I've found is along the wrist. Place both your hands palms up in front of you. Now take one of your hands and place the index and middle finger of that hand on the outside of the wrist of the opposite hand. The fingers should lie together on the opposite wrist in line with the index finger. Feel for a pulse. When you find a pulse, count the number of beats in 10 seconds and then multiply by 6. If you want to be more accurate, count beats for 15 seconds and multiply by 4, or count for 30 seconds and multiply by 2 or simply count for 60 seconds. The more time you count for, the more accurate your measure.

Maximum heart rate (MHR)

For men: (220−your Age). If you are a male, age 45. Your MHR=220-45=175

For women: (226−your Age). If you are a female, age 45. Your MHR=226-45=181

❖ HEALTH ZONE:

This amounts to 50 to 60% of your maximum heart rate (MHR).
Within this pulse range, the cardiovascular system will be invigorated. This range is particularly suitable for beginners.

❖ FAT BURNING ZONE:

This amounts to 60 to 70% of your maximum heart rate (MHR).
Within this pulse range, most calories from fat are burned.

❖ AEROBIC ZONE:

This amounts to 70 to 80% of your maximum heart rate (MHR).
Within this pulse range, carbohydrates and fats are burned for power production in the muscle cells.

❖ ANAEROBIC ZONE:

This amounts to 80 to 90% of your maximum heart rate (MHR).
Within this pulse range, the body cannot cover the oxygen demand any longer. This range is for the development of power and muscle mass.

❖ RED ZONE:

This amounts to 90 to 100% of your maximum heart rate (MHR).
This pulse range should be handled with caution. It is dangerous for
beginners and can be harmful for the heart.

Fat Blasting and Toning Exercises

These exercises are done periodically and targets specific muscle
groups, so there are effective exercises for each group. Always
start with stretches to warm up the muscles. You may need to
invest in some weights or equipment. To effectively tone your
muscles, you will need to determine the maximum weight you can
correctly lift once without repetition. This becomes what is known
as your 1 range of motion (1 RM). Then determine what 65% of
your 1 RM is. For example. If your 1 RM=10 kg, then your 65% is
6.5kg.

This weight is what your target muscle group should correctly
lift for 10–15 times. This forms a set. This means a set is made of
10–15 movements or repetitions (reps). Then do 3 sets with a 30
to 60 seconds rest period between each set. Please do not change
the weight for that particular exercise. After a period of regular
exercise, see if your 1RM has increased. For variations of these
exercises, consult your muscle magazine or gym instructor.

Day One (3 sets of 15 repetitions, rest for 60 seconds)
Chest Exercises: Inclined Dumbbell Press, Inclined Dumbbell Fly
Shoulder Exercises: Seated Dumbbell Lateral Raise, Dumbbell Shoulder Press
Back Exercises: Dead Lift, Double Dumbbell Row
Arm Exercises: Dumbbell Curls, Triceps Pull downs
Cardio-Jog-Sprint Cycles

Day Two—Rest

Day Three (3 sets of 15 repetitions, rest for 60 seconds)
Abdominal Exercises: Crunches, Inclined Knee Raises
Cardio-Jog-Sprint Cycles

Day Four—Rest

Day Five (3 sets of 15 repetitions, rest for 60 seconds)
Quadriceps Exercises: Leg Extensions, Barbell Squats
Hamstring Exercises: Unilateral Leg Curls
Calf Exercises: Calf Raises
Cardio-Jog-Sprint Cycles

Muscles Exercises

These exercises are done periodically. These exercises target specific muscle groups, so there is an effective exercise for each group. Always start with stretches to warm up the muscles. You may need to invest in some weights or equipment. To effectively build your muscles, you will need to determine the maximum weight you can correctly lift once without repetition and work those muscles to the point of failure (the point when you can no longer lift the weight). This is about your 1RM weight. Determine what 80% of your 1RM is. For example, if your 1RM=10 kg then your 80% is 8.0kg.

For the first set, you lift 8 kg for 12–15 times. Rest for 60 to 90 seconds then increase the weights to about 85% of your 1RM and lift for 8–10 times then rest. Continue increasing the weights to 90% and lift for 6–8 times then rest. Continue increasing weights and decreasing the number of repetitions, until that muscle group reaches failure, which should be close to the weight of your 1RM. Failure is the point where you can no longer execute the lift, because the muscles are fatigued. For variations of these exercises, consult your muscle magazine or gym instructor.

Day One (3 sets of repetitions, rest for 90 seconds)
Chest Exercises: Inclined Dumbbell Press, Inclined Dumbbell Fly
Shoulder Exercises: Seated Dumbbell Lateral raise, Dumbbell Shoulder Press
Back Exercises: Dead Lift, Double Dumbbell Row
Arm Exercises: Dumbbell Curls, Triceps Pull downs
Cardio-Jog-Sprint Cycles

Day Two—Rest

Day Three (3 sets of repetitions, rest for 90 seconds)
Abdominal Exercises: Crunches, Inclined Knee Raises
Cardio-Jog-Sprint Cycles

Day Four—Rest

Day Five (3 sets of repetitions, rest for 90 seconds)
Quadriceps Exercises: Leg Extensions, Barbell Squats
Hamstring Exercises: Unilateral Leg Curls
Calf Exercises: Calf Raises
Cardio-Jog-Sprint Cycles

Losing Those Last Few Pounds

After losing weight steadily, you may get to a stage known as the "plateau," where the weight loss stops.

This situation is common among those who are classified as endomorphs. It is accepted that people come in one of three body types. These are the endomorphs, ectomorphs and mesomorphs.

Ectomorphs are naturally skinny. They appear to have a metabolic system that burns fat no matter what they eat. They easily lose weight but have great difficulty in building muscle. I recommend they add protein shakes to their diet and exercise regime.

Mesomorphs are those who easily gain and lose weight. To lose weight they only need to eat right and exercise right.

Endomorphs are those whose body system loves to store body fat. They easily put on weight and often find it hard to lose weight or they may lose weight steadily for a while then the weight loss stops for no apparent reason. For endomorphs, the solution lies in a more stringent form of attack on the body fat. To lose those last few pounds, endomorphs may need to switch to a strict vegetable, fruit and nut diet for a while. No more lean meats until they get to their desired weight, then they can resume eating lean meats. Also, they will need to increase the aerobic level of the exercises they do. These combinations are guaranteed to blast away those last stubborn inches of body fat.

If you cannot bear to stop eating meats, then you might need to add thermogenic or fat-burner pills to your nutrition and exercise regime. A word of caution! Do not go for unbranded manufacturers, some of these pills are very potent and can hurt you if taken inappropriately. Always start with a minimum dosage and see if there are any unpleasant side effects. The pills are also the combinations of many properties, so they do not affect everyone the same way. You will have to determine which pill best suits your body chemistry. I recommend using pills produced from natural sources, however, if in doubt, always consult your physician.

Finally, your mind can play a vital in getting rid of those last few pounds. Talk to yourself. Tell yourself how proud you are of what it has achieved so far, and that you are confident it can lose the remaining few pounds. Keep doing this even when you are not exercising.

Recipes

STIR FRY BEANS

Ingredients
1 cup beans
Soy sauce
Tomatoes, onions, peppers

Directions
Wash and cook beans. Splash soy sauce to coat beans. Stir continuously. Add sesame seeds, strips of onions, tomatoes or peppers and cook for 7 to 10 minutes.

GBEGIRI (BEAN SOUP)

Ingredients
1 cup beans
3 oz tomato paste
Chilli powder to taste
Food seasoning cubes or granules to taste
Salt to taste
2tsp olive oil
0.5 cup chopped fresh onion-
(Optional) 300 grams mackerel fish

Directions
Soak the beans for about 5 minutes, remove the skin very well and cook the until it is very soft. Blend the cooked beans into a very creamy soup. Add as much water as you prefer; do not cover the pot again from this point. Clean your fish and cut into desired sizes. Add all ingredients and the fish into the cream and cook until the fish is properly cooked. Do not to cover the pot after you have added water and other ingredients to avoid foaming.

MOIN MOIN (BEAN PUDDING)
Ingredients
Beans
Bouillon cubes
Salt water
Cooked liver Hard boiled egg (Optional) fish
Palm or olive oil
Jalapeno and chilli peppers
Onion

Directions
Wash beans and soak for about 15 minutes. Rub beans between palms until skin comes off. Add beans, onions, water and peppers and blend together until smooth. Pour out the paste into a bowl and add the chopped up egg, salt and food seasoning cubes to taste and the oil. Mix in one direction until every thing is mixed and the colour is even.
Pour into a greased baking dish and cover with foil or film. Put into a pre-heated oven at the 220-degree mark and let it cook for about 20 to 30 minutes.

EFO RIRO (SPINACH STEW)
Ingredients
Spinach
Pepper
Tomatoes
Salt to taste
Ground cinnamon
Extra virgin olive or vegetable oil
(Optional) fried fish, cooked liver, kponmo (softened cow skin)

Directions
Steam spinach and set. Dice all the vegetables and stir-fry for 2 minutes. Add the steamed spinach and allow to simmer for 1 minute. Add the ground cinnamon and allow setting. Serve hot with grilled mackerel (optional).

EWEDU STEW
Ingredients
200g ewedu leaves
1 tsp of potash (optional)
A pinch of salt

1 seasoning cube
Stew

Directions
Pick the leaves (no steam allowed) of the ewedu and wash properly. Boil the ewedu leaves in a pot for about 15 mins. Add the potash to help in softening it, a pinch of salt and the seasoning cube. When soft, you can whisk it or you blend it with a blender. Serve it with stew.

AKARA (FRIED BEAN BALLS)
Ingredients
2 cups beans, peeled
Salt to taste
1 seasoning cube
Pepper to taste
1 onion bulb
Vegetable oil for deep frying

Directions
Grind the peeled beans with the onions to obtain a very thick paste. Mix properly with a cube of maggi, salt and pepper. Scoop into balls and deep-fry the beans balls. Serve fresh and hot.

JOLLOF BEANS (BEAN PORRIDGE)
Ingredients
400 g beans
2 onion bulbs
Chilli pepper to taste
2 seasoning cubes
1 cup stock (optional)
1 cup palm or olive oil
½ cup crayfish (optional)
Salt to taste

Directions
Wash the beans properly and cook with all the onions for about 45 mins. Add the chilli pepper, food seasoning cubes, stock, crayfish and palm oil. Allow cooking for another 5 mins. Stir properly and add salt to taste. Serve as desired.

AFANG STEW
Ingredients
Afang leaves, pounded
Waterleaf or spinach
1 kg meat/chicken/goat meat
Rich meat stock
300 g softened stockfish
Dried fish
200 g kponmo (softened cow skin)
4 cups periwinkle (optional)
6 chilli peppers
1 cup Crayfish, ground (optional)
2 seasoning cubes to taste
2 cups palm or olive oil
1 onion bulb

Directions
Cook the meat until soft, add the stockfish, dried fish and kpomo. Cook until you have about one cup of stock water in the pot. Add the waterleaf and cook for about 3 mins. Add the Afang leaves, crayfish and the oil. Cook for about 5 mins with the food seasoning cubes and pepper. Add salt to taste.

OGBONO STEW

Ingredients
3 cups of stock
1 kg meat
1 cup pumpkin leaves or bitter leaf, nicely chopped
1 cup ogbono, ground
400 g dried fish (optional)
400 g stockfish (optional)
200 g kponmo, (softened cow skin)
1 cup crayfish, ground (optional)
2 cups shelled periwinkle (optional)
8 chilli peppers to taste
2 seasoning cubes
1 cup palm or olive oil
1 onion
Salt to taste

Directions
Wash all the ingredients properly. Season and boil the meat to obtain the broth. When the meat is almost soft, add the stockfish and kpomo. In a different pot, boil your periwinkle in salt water and wash properly. Add about 6 cups of water when the stockfish, meat and kpomo are soft. Bring to a boil. Add the ogbono, perewinkle and oil and cook for about 5 mins. Add the chopped pumpkin leaves or bitterleaf, crayfish and seasoning cubes. Boil for another 3 mins and add salt to taste.

OKRA SOUP
Ingredients
1 kg beef/chicken/goat meat
400 g okra, chopped or pounded
400 g dried fish (optional)
300 g stockfish (optional)
300 g kponmo (softened cow skin) (optional)
1 ½ cups crayfish (ground) (optional)

8 chilli pepper
2 cups erwinkle (optional)
3 seasoning cubes
2 cups palm or vegetable oil
1 onion
Salt to taste

Directions
Wash all the ingredients properly. Season and boil the meat to obtain the broth. When the meat is almost soft, add the stockfish and kpomo. Boil your periwinkle in salt water and wash properly. Add about 6 cups of water when the stockfish, meat and kpomo are soft. Bring to a boil. Add the grated okra and palm oil and cook for about 5 mins. Boil for another 3 mins and add salt to taste.

VEGETABLE SAUCE
Ingredients
100 g tomatoes, sliced
1 large onion, sliced
1 seasoning cube
½ tsp curry powder
A dash of thyme

A dash of oregano
Chilli pepper to taste
1 red pepper, sliced
1 green pepper, sliced
200 g carrots, sliced
50 g peas
½ cup vegetable oil for stirring
200 g diced steamed meat
Salt to taste

Directions
Put a pan on heat and add the onions. Add the steamed meat and tomatoes. Fry with low heat for about 5 mins. Pour every other vegetable and stir-fry. Add the spices and salt. Serve as desired.

MEAT STEW
Ingredients
1 kg beef/goat/turkey/fish/chicken
Stock, as much as desired consistency
4 cups blended tomatoes
Chilli pepper to taste
1 paprika bulb
2 onion bulbs, chopped
1 tsp curry
½ tsp thyme
1 garlic clove, crushed
1 tsp freshly grated ginger
1 food seasoning cube
1 cup vegetable oil

Directions
Season meat properly to get the stock. When cooked, you could fry or grill the meat. Pour the vegetable oil into a pot and place on heat. Throw in the chopped onions when the oil is hot. Pour the blended tomatoes into the pot and allow to cook for about 10 mins. Pour in the stock and cook further. Add the seasoning cube, ginger, crushed garlic, curry and thyme. Cook for another 20 mins. Add the meat and salt to taste.

PEPPER SOUPS
Ingredients
1 kg goat meat, chicken, cow tail, bush meat, assorted meats or fish

2 food seasoning cubes
1 onion bulb
Pepper to taste
½ tsp ground ehuru seeds (optional)
Salt to taste
Mint leaf (optional)
Traditional aromatic pepper soup spices (optional)

Directions
Season the meat properly with the ingredients. Add about 5 cups of water. Cook till the meat is soft. Add the peppersoup spices if necessary. Add the scent leaf. Salt to taste.

EDIKANG IKONG STEW
Ingredients
Pumpkin leaves
Water leaves
Beef, kponmo(softened cow skin) and dry fish
Pepper, salt and ground crayfish to taste
30 cl. palm or olive oil
1 cup periwinkle (optional)
2 medium onions bulbs
3 food seasoning cubes

Directions
Wash and cut the pumpkin and water leaves into tiny pieces. Put them in separate sieves to drain out all the water. Cut the kponmo into small pieces. Cook the beef, kponmo(softened cow skin) and the dry fish with the 2 bulbs of diced onions and the 3 food seasoning cubes with as little quantity of water as possible. Add some oil, the crayfish and pepper and leave to boil for about 10 mins. Add the periwinkle and waterleaves and leave to cook for another 5 mins. Now add the pumpkin leaves and salt to taste. Stir the contents of the pot and turn off the heat. Cover the pot and leave to stand for about 5 mins

HUMUS
Ingredients
1 can garbanzo beans or cooked chickpeas
2 tbsp extra virgin olive oil
1 clove garlic

Juice of 1 small lemon
2-3 tbsp Tahini sauce
Salt to taste

Directions
Drain a third of the water from the can of garbanzo beans or cooked chick peas into a bowl. Keep the drained water. Blend, the garbanzo beans or cooked chickpeas with rest of the ingredients and can water. Blend for about 1 to 2 minutes till a smooth, slightly fluid paste is formed. Sprinkle paprika. Serve with flat bread.

Conclusions

I hope this book motivates you to lose the weight forever.
I have no regrets and neither will you.
I just wished that someone else had written this book twenty years ago.

Acknowledgements

I would like to acknowledge these special people in my life: my wife (Bolaji), my daughter (Simi), my two boys (Demi and Dami) and my dad (Ajani Ekun)

THIS BOOK IS DEDICATED TO GOD THE ALMIGHTY